—

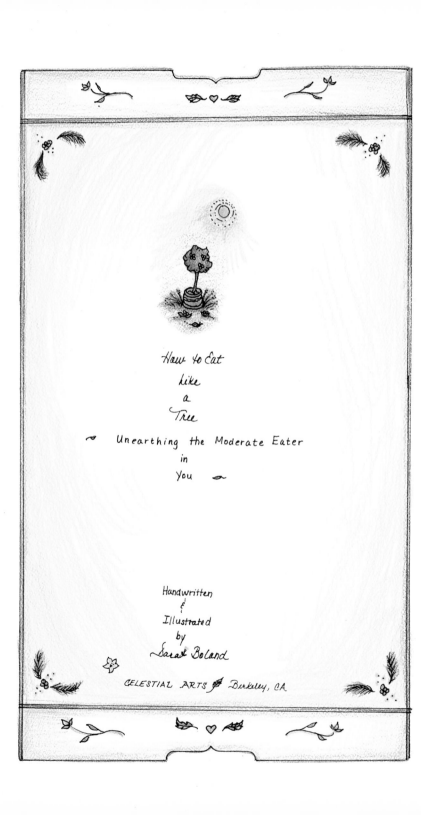

How to Eat

Like

a

Tree

Unearthing the Moderate Eater

in

You

Handwritten
&
Illustrated
by
Sarah Boland

CELESTIAL ARTS · Berkeley, CA

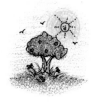

Celestial Arts
P. O. Box 7123
Berkeley, California 94707

Distributed in Canada by Ten Speed Canada, in the United Kingdom and Europe by Airlift Books, in New Zealand by Southern Publishers Group, in Australia by Simon & Schuster Australia, in South Africa by Real Books, and in Singapore, Malaysia, Hong Kong, and Thailand by Berkeley Books.

Cover illustrations by Sara Boland
Cover design by Libby Oda

Library of Congress Catalog Card Number:
99-75064
A Heart & Star Book
First printing, 2000
Printed in Hong Kong

1 2 3 4 5 6 7 — 04 03 02 01 00

To
Nannie
&
Boppie

who
saved
my
life
&
taught
me
how
to
love...

♥

...UNCONDITIONALLY...

and...

To
David

without
whose support
this book
never could have
been
written
&
illustrated
by
moi

~❀~

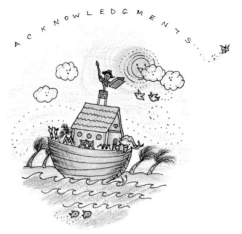

A C K N O W L E D G M E N T S . . .

From the bottom of my heart el want to thank Alice Martell, my agent and the angel who believed in my project through it all:

el thank you, Alice.

Kathryn Ettinger and Jo Ann Deck and Veronica Randall at Celestial Arts: thank you for your patient kindness with me, at all times (even when el was freaking out).

Thanks so much to my friends and family who were there when el needed them: Betsy, Stephanie, Joyce, Mom, Michael & Matthew, Mark & Krista, Margaret, Mollie & Abby (who show us why being girls is so great). And el want to thank Dad for bringing home my inspiration: my first Joan Walsh Anglund book. Woody & Rebecca ~ thanks, too!

And Boppie, your persistence and exuberance kept me going with this well past the time el "should have" given up on it. And Nannie, for your love ~ regardless

Thanks to Rhonda Mann at the North Carolina State University Women's Center, who asked me to do the workshops there. This book was written for all who have our questions.

Thanks, David!

Peace.

Thanks, Bill at MBE!

TABLE OF CONTENTS

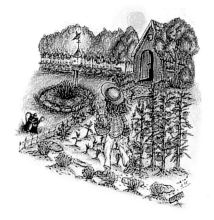

"When I go into my garden with a spade,
and dig a bed, I feel such an exhilaration
& health that I discover that I have been
defrauding myself all this time in letting
others do for me what I should have done
with my own hands.

~RALPH WALDO EMERSON
Man the Reformer

I

the uintroduction :

As a part
of Nature, you have
within you an inherent
I N C L I N A T I O N
to be moderate and achieve
. . B   A   L   A   N   C   E
. . . . in all things.

You have within you a natural
eating ideal based on the innate
signals your body wants to give to
your mind with regard to energy
and eating and living

♡ S   A   T   I   S   F   A   C   T   I   O   N .

It is this communication
process
that will guide you
to
your
own
UNIQUE
ideal
BODY - MIND
CONDITION
~ weight · wise and otherwise ~ ...

Most of all, this process you are about to
uncover from within you WILL MAINTAIN THAT
UNIQUE IDEAL.

It just needs to be
unearthed . . .

Now let's go ····· →

I

For you, dear reader...

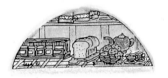

If
you
garden

or just love to see
beautiful flowers & sunsets,
or if you like to take long walks...

If
you
want more balance
in

~ your days

~ your priorities

~ the foods you put into your
body...

If you yearn for a simple life
governed by a natural love for
yourself; for your body; for all
those people, places & pastimes
that mean the most to you ....

This book was handwritten
for you ♡

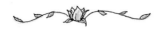

The very essence
of
Balance
is
the equal distribution
of both
the positive
and the negative

that exists
in every area
of your life,
not only in your menu.

Food may be love
at the moment,
but it doesn't have to be
the only
~ or the best ~
Love
there is.

You decide ; you make
the choice.

Start to love your body as it is
right now
and put the wheels
of
"Positivity"
into motion.

Easier said than done, right?

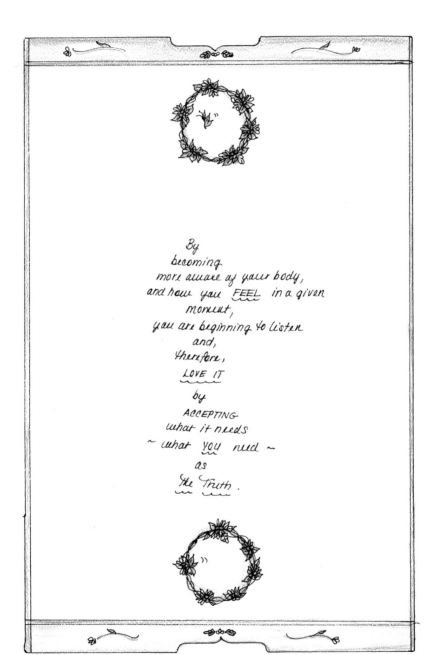

By
becoming
more aware of your body,
and how you FEEL in a given
moment,
you are beginning to listen
and,
therefore,
LOVE IT
by
ACCEPTING
what it needs
~ what YOU need ~
as
the Truth.

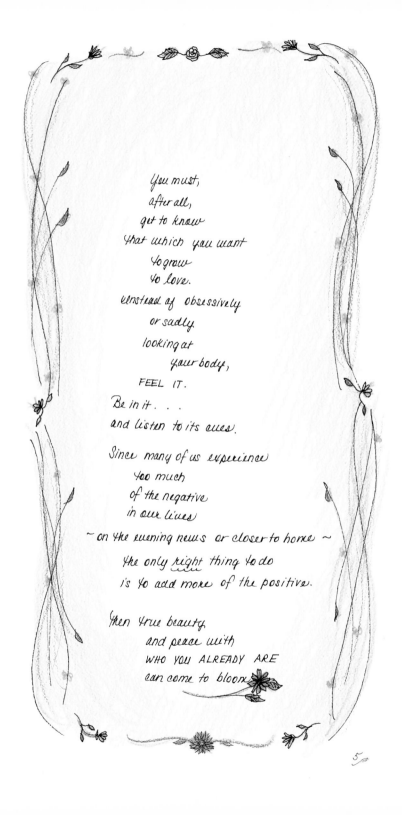

You must,
after all,
get to know
that which you want
to grow
to love.

Instead of obsessively
or sadly
looking at
your body,
FEEL IT.
Be in it . . .
and listen to its cues.

Since many of us experience
too much
of the negative
in our lives
~ on the evening news or closer to home ~
the only right thing to do
is to add more of the positive.

Then true beauty
and peace with
WHO YOU ALREADY ARE
can come to bloom.

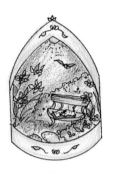

Beauty
is,
after all,
a balance in
and of
itself,
from the inside to the outside
and back again
to
the
beginning...
to who and what you
were meant to be
in the very first place.
Let
the
beauty
~ the balance ~
begin ....

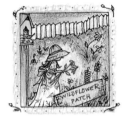

"If a man be weary....
there is no better place in the world
to recreate himself than a garden."

~ WILLIAM COLES
Art of Simpling

II

MY PERSONAL VIEW

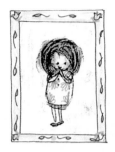

Mother Nature is the greatest
moderator of them all.

    I realized this several
years ago, after living more than
half my life with disordered eating.

    At 12 I was hospitalized for
the first time for anorexia ~ I
weighed 39 pounds. Twelve years
later I was out of college with my
degree and a habit of snack food
binge eating that left me well
over 100 pounds heavier. (I'm not
sure how much I weighed since I had thrown
my scale out in frustration).

    Throwing out the scale was the best thing I ever did.
After all, Mother Nature doesn't count, nor does she keep track.
She goes by INSTINCT, by FEELING, by all the things we're
left with when the layers of false food conditioning and
"shoulds" are brushed away.

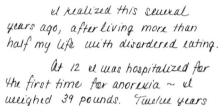

She goes   by her own

INNER   TRUTH

And now,   so can we . . .   ⟶

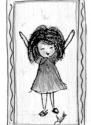

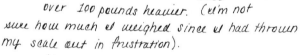

IMAGINE...

eating
like you meant it,
like you treasure it,
each bite at a time.

imagine
eating for your exact body's needs
and not really knowing it.

imagine cravings were good things*

How do you get there,
    back to
one-at-a-time cookie jar treats...
to apples so perfect
that you crunch into them
and let the juice run down your chin
with abandon....

        to a place
            where ice cream sundaes
can peacefully   coexist with

        brilliantly hued
                carrot sticks
                ....

and where a craving for
    z u c c h i n i
rivals that for pepperoni
            PIZZA   ?

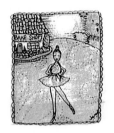

How do you get back
to a body
that loves food
and
to a mind
that says, "Okay,"
~ because it really, really is ~
even on the first day of bathing suit
season?

Imagine
u n e a r t h i n g
YOUR NATURAL EATING
n i c h e.

Imagine
living at a weight perfect
for your body type.

Imagine...

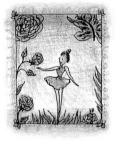

E A T I N G

as
Mother Nature
meant
you
to.

Imagine

eating

like

a

tree....

R e m e m b e r . . .

back at the
beginning,

when you were a kid ?

NOT   JUST   EATING...

but licking, chewing, scraping the creme
out of the inside of an Oreo
& grinning a brown-speckled grin ?

Back when you "saved room" for the Mister Softy
ice cream cone after dinner...
the thrill of hearing canned ice cream truck music
off in the distance,
standing out at the curb
with friends,
each trying to guess which block he was on ?

Remember...

the aroma of a hot pizza
in a soggy box
on those nights when Mom
was too rushed to cook ?

Remember...

the
nip
in
the
air...

while picking pumpkins
in a big field
on burgundy- and gold-colored
autumn days...

trick-or-treating with your little sister
("Hold her hand, now!" Mom would warn)

...not   only   for   the   candy

but

for   the   costume

for the one night when you were allowed
outside after dark,

running from house to house
on familiar daytime streets....

Remember?
the sweetness of a McIntosh
plucked
from a basin of icy-cold, apple-bobbing
water?

Or...

the one time in your life, perhaps,

when you could remember what you ate

~ even now ~

so many years later ?

Peanut butter and grape jelly sandwiches
on
W o n d e r   B r e a d
in
waxed little baggies ...

shiny red apples or oranges you'd
peel, only to shoot juice at your
pals across the table ...

Miniature cartons of milk ...
and peanut butter tastes
lingering in your mouth
in Science class,

oddly mixed with the dry scent
of wooden pencil shavings and
your teacher's

favorite perfume ?

Picture the way it was
the way it
...smelled...
... felt...
... tasted...
back then ....

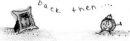

Back when
    eating meant something...
but not everything.

When food was your fun friend,
not your shoulder to cry on,
    to shout at, curse, or fear.

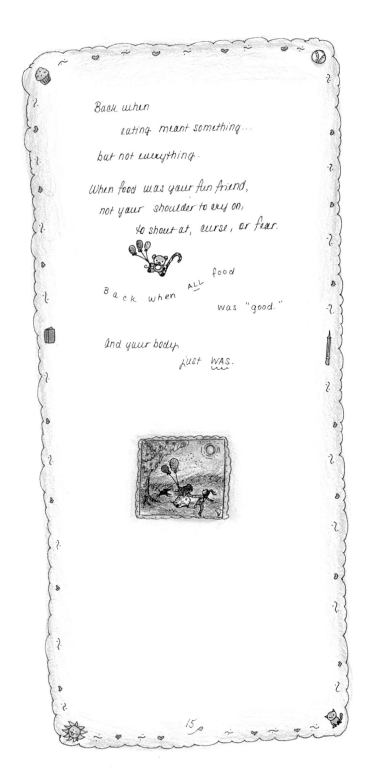

Back when ALL food
            was "good."

And your body
        just WAS.

Kids eat like trees.
So do naturally lean people.
  (Watch them sometime...)

They eat FOR their bodies,
    not in spite of them.

They eat for all the positive,
        good reasons:

· · energy ! · ·
            TASTE
              &
Satisfaction

They eat
to maintain
their energy level
    ~
not to jumpstart
    or sedate it.

They eat to live and they live to eat...
along with a lot of other things

                as
                well...

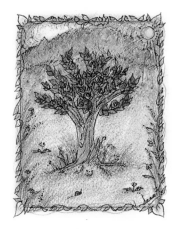

"And out of the ground
the Lord God
caused to grow
every tree
that is pleasing to the sight,
and
good for food...."

~ GENESIS 2:9

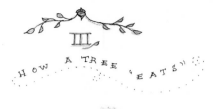

III

HOW A TREE 'EATS'

Trees, of course, don't "eat" the way we do. But considering a tree's roots, not to mention its trunk, leaves, and branches, are literally surrounded by "tree food" all day, why then don't they, like us humans, overdo it, at least once in a while?

The answer is two-fold:

(1)   They **do** "overdo it" ~

   once in a while
. . . .

~ and ~

(2)   Most of the time they are too busy

KEEPING THE BALANCE

~ inside and outside of themselves ~

going.

Nature calls this HOMEOSTASIS.
On trees this is instinctual.

On humans, who are bombarded with

false messages

that cloud our natural~born
instinct to eat and to move

well for our bodies'
and our minds'

personal sense of peace,

this may need to be unearthed... →

18

"HOMEOSTATIC EATING"

Humans

call this balance

~ this homeostasis

on a human level ~

Moderation in all things

~ including food

~ including the weight
it leaves us with

and

~~~ m o s t of all ~~~

THE DAILY HABITS WE USE

to keep

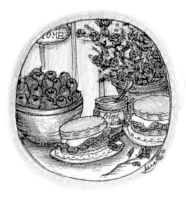

us there.

Trees eat:

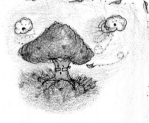

1. Selectively

2. Slowly, in small increments

3. Always with the environment 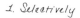 around them and what it will bear.

4. What they need

5. When they need it
   (if possible)

6. For their unique energy
   (& species') needs

~ A N D ~

7. As nourishment ~ for themselves and, in turn, for the environment around them.

Trees "eat" from the inside out
         and from
     the outside in.

THEY TAKE IN ALL THAT THEY NEED
         TO GROW
         & TO FLOURISH
& let out all the "stuff" that they do not.

...IT...

just so happens
that we
~ and all living creatures ~
need
"that stuff"
to
live:

A I R,

cool shade,

solid ground

(erosion - proof)...

and so much more.

Trees are WHOLE SYSTEMS
unto
themselves.

They give to the world around them,
the world they are a part of,
and they take what they need
in order to survive
and to be, beautifully,
their own kind
of tree.

For trees, this comes naturally.

That's what it means to eat like a tree.

Ideally, humans would follow
their natures
in
the same way.

The problem is,
in all our intelligence, with our technological &
medical advances,
we've forgotten where we came from.

We've forgotten
how to eat
by simply listening to our bodies,
by "hearing" and addressing all of our cravings

... not only for food,
     but for other things as well.
(When was the last time you got
enough sleep
EVERY NIGHT
... for a whole week straight ?)...

Cravings
~ whether for sleep or certain foods
     or companionship
     or just plain peace ~

are good things.

They are the Voice
of our own unique message center
that will guide us
toward the process
that creates a balanced body
and
a balanced life ....

IV

THE 7 STEPS

The seven steps we are
about to take to unearth your
eating and lifestyle peace are ~
not ironically ~ identical to those
you would take in transplanting a
new tree.

   Most importantly, taking these
seven steps will enable you to enjoy
living with food IN YOUR BODY, as you
once may have done as a child ... as you
were meant to do as the beautifully UNIQUE
person that you are today.

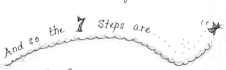

And so the 7 Steps are ....

1. Consider the climate.
2. Choose the site.
3. Break ground.
4. Dig shallow and wide.
5. Prepare the soil.
6. Add organic matter.
7. Mulch to protect.

(huh?)

... grab a shovel and .... let's go .... !

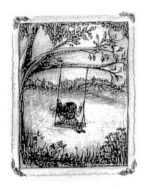

" A garden
         without trees
    scarcely deserves
         to be called
              a
            Garden. "

— CANON   HENRY   ELLACOMBE
    In a Gloucestershire Garden

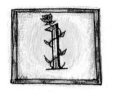

Consider the Climate.

> "It is the disease
> of not listening...
> that I am troubled with."
>
> — WILLIAM SHAKESPEARE

LOOK OUTSIDE.

The first clues as to why you don't eat well for your body frame are right outside your personal windows: your eyes and your ears.

Look around. Listen.

What's going on around you at this moment? What went on around you earlier this day?

~ Is work too hectic for your nerves?

~ Have you "outgrown" your job, or any other role you've taken in life?

~ Is the dog neglected?

~ Are you not getting enough time with the kids?

Are you saying, "Okay, I'll do it"... way too much?

25

Now <u>look inside.</u>

Why?

Why do you believe, on some level, that you alone cannot say, "No," once in a while to everything "Out there" (work, home demands, and other obligations), and say, "Yes," instead to what you are crying out for <u>FROM THE INSIDE</u>?

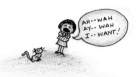

Too often, we blame ourselves for not being able (or willing, or both) to keep up with all the constants out there, but in reality it is our own personal perception that shapes the climate we are left with "in here."

Moderate living is a form of self-love. WE MUST BE WILLING TO TAKE SOME TIME TO LISTEN TO OURSELVES ONCE IN A WHILE ~ SO LISTENING FROM <u>WITHIN</u> becomes the habit we live with, constantly.

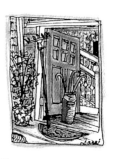

Look inside ...
    to how and when and
    how often you take care of You
    just as you would any other
    Loved One.

HOW OFTEN DO YOU ASK YOURSELF FIRST,

    "elf I could have [or do ... or eat]
    anything right now, what would it be?"

        NO NEED TO REDO
        YOUR LIFE RIGHT NOW...
    WE   ARE   ONLY
                PLANTING   SEEDS

                    for improvement later.

AN EXAMPLE OF PEEKING
INSIDE...

~ think of how often you indulge
    ♡ in a warm bath
    ♡ in a good book
    ♡ in time to listen to an
audiotape that soothes you
    ♡ in a hobby that interests you,
        just for the fun of it.

How often do you simply let yourself

       P L A Y

        ?

Are all of your thrills laced
with chocolate?

No wonder the scales
          are
        imbalanced....

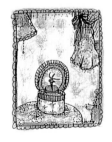

~ look inside.

~ LISTEN to your wants
your desires
your cravings.

DON'T WORRY ABOUT MAJOR CHANGES...

Just
see
more, for now.

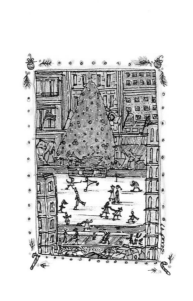

" When it gets dark enough,
you can see the stars."

CHARLES A. BEARD

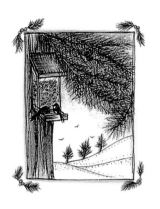

LOOK INSIDE ~
around the food instead.

What are <u>ALL THOSE OTHER THINGS</u> in your life
that cause you to overeat?
things like:

☞ those past experiences that prevent you from
loving yourself enough to give yourself the
gift of self-care ...

☞ those outside triggers that unconsciously
signal you to overeat ...

☞ all those other aspects of "climate" that
can leave you with a big, empty hole to fill ~
with too much food...
or the wrong kinds of food.

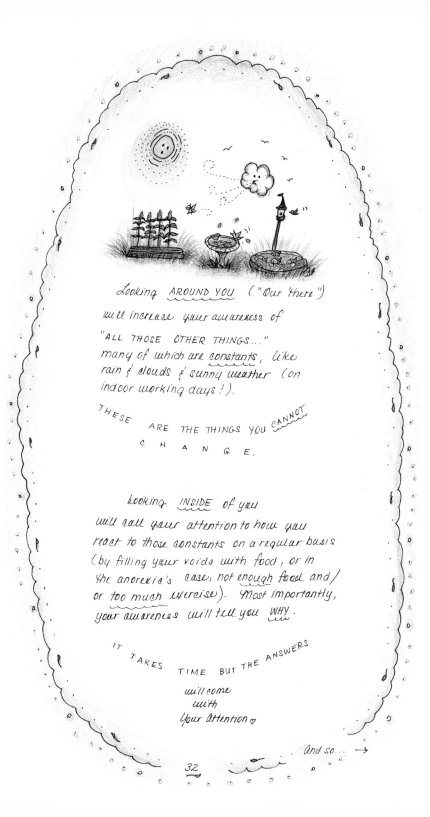

Looking AROUND YOU ("Out there")
will increase your awareness of
"ALL THOSE OTHER THINGS..."
many of which are constants, like
rain & clouds & sunny weather (on
indoor working days!).

THESE ARE THE THINGS YOU CANNOT
C H A N G E.

Looking INSIDE of you
will call your attention to how you
react to those constants on a regular basis
(by filling your voids with food, or in
the anorexic's case, not enough food and/
or too much exercise). Most importantly,
your awareness will tell you WHY.

IT TAKES TIME BUT THE ANSWERS
will come
with
your attention ♡

And so... →

32

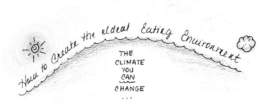

How to Create the eldeal Eating Environment

THE
CLIMATE
YOU
CAN
CHANGE
...

1. Set the table, with napkin, fork, spoon & knife ~ even if it is only at your desk or kitchen counter. Bring the knife to the table, and the spoon, too, at first, even if you don't think you'll need them. Kinder eating may require more "tools" than you're used to....

2. Choose your food wisely. By "wisely" I mean "consciously." Always try to remember to ask yourself before you eat ~ even if it's only a quick snack ~ what it is you REALLY want to eat, and...

~ then try to get it (or a second best choice, or third, if need be). Don't worry about fat content or nutritional value just yet... and if this is next to impossible for you, PRETEND it doesn't matter at this moment. (A doctor's warning or allergy, of course, precludes this step ... but choose from what is reasonably AVAILABLE to you....)

What we are doing is . . . .

PLANTING HEALTHY SEEDS.

Simply begin the lifelong habit
of feeding
your body
your taste buds
&
your craving mind.

(We're starting with food since we

like
it
very much)

...

And final step :

3. Eat slowly and savor every bite
~ every CALORIE, if you must think of
it that way (we know we did!).

~ Remind yourself that, like trees
and birds and plants and little children,
you deserve to eat, and to relish each
and every bite.

For trees and birds and plants and little children, this comes

Naturally...

and hasn't been wiped out
by
infinite
"Shoulds"
(and "should 'nots"!).

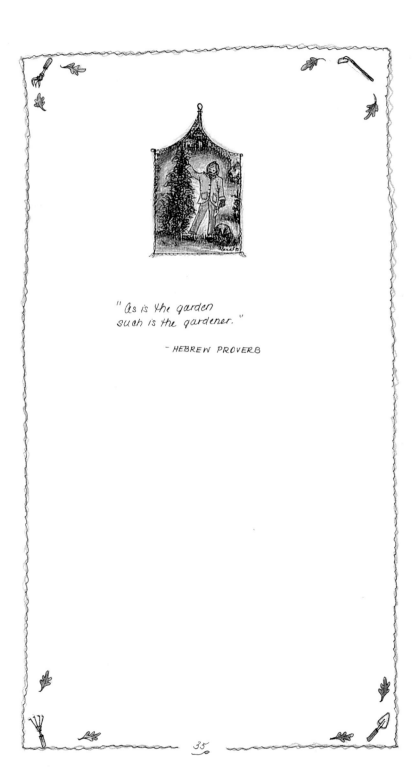

" As is the garden
such is the gardener. "

— HEBREW PROVERB

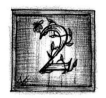

Choose the Site.

the
site
of becoming moderate
with all things ~ including
food and weight ~ is not your mouth,
nor your hands, nor your plate....

the
site
of
MODERATE EATING
is
the
mind...

Your
mind.

After all, every action ~
however small ~
is
preceded by a thought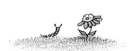

When you first
were learning
how to walk, it took
all the thought and energy
you could give it.

IF YOU GARDEN...

~ When you planted your first flower in a pot
or in a flower bed you may have struggled with
how to plant it properly. The thought of
planting it intrigued you, and so you went about
discovering the necessary steps required to do so.

And,

as all gardeners know,
you learned ~ and continue
to learn
with each seed
each plant
each flower
and tree
~
by trial and error.

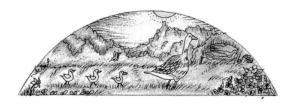

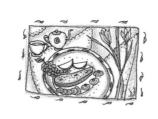

Well,

we've TRIED

to become content

with

ourselves

through perfecting

our bodies

by

dieting... starving... depriving

and

we've

ERRED.

Perfection isn't the point. Balance is...

leave your plate and your cupboards
and your clothes closet alone.

Let's look INSIDE, to the source
of our discomfort and discontent.

Let's go beneath the dirt,
to the roots of good eating:

the habits

that run it

❀ and help it to grow.... ❀

❀ The Mind is the Source ❀

MODERATION IS A
HABIT

Habits are processes we have
come to repeat because trial and error
have proven them to WORK FOR US.

Habits ~ eating and otherwise ~
begin with THOUGHTS. Sometimes these
thoughts are deeply buried in our
minds because of that lovely......
mental phenomenon known as...

AUTOMATIC PILOT

How many times have you eaten
a whole bag of chips ~ or anything ~
UNCONSCIOUSLY ?

On the flip side, how many times
have you overdone it in the garden,
or in your work, or on a breathless day of
fun-filled vacationing? Your body automatically
moves to keep pace with your enthusiasm ~
and tells you about it the next stiff-backed
morning...........

So it is with MODERATE EATING!

~ It's something that starts small,
like a bulb in the dirt in early Spring

~ It's something that grows
with and for and BECAUSE OF the environment
around it.

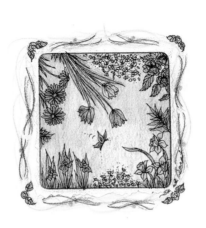

~ It needs "feeding" to grow, but...

~ Soon it becomes its own "automatic pilot,"

and finally...

~ It's this "automatic pilot" that will
maintain our moderate weight
and more balanced life.

~•~

Many of us are in the very NEGATIVE
habit of WORRYING ~ about our weight
or what we are NOT eating or doing "right."
Energy used for worrying is WASTED.
Begin in small ways to direct your precious
energy in each given day toward something
you prefer... for your body, mind & soul.
~ Pretty soon that "automatic pilot" will kick in!

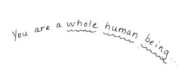

You are a whole human being...

∽ A WHOLE SYSTEM, TOO ∾

with many different
physical, psychological, and
spiritual needs.

These needs and what fills
them are "ALL THOSE OTHER THINGS."

And...

in order for any ACTION
or PROCESS to become YOUR HABIT,
it must work FOR you on one or all
of these highly personal LEVELS.

Whatever hasn't worked for you
in the past was starving you on one
~ or all ~ of these levels, and so
you dropped it like a slug stuck on
a garden glove!

(ICK!)

And so ...

the question is this:

What about _your_ environment
is starving one or some or ALL THOSE
OTHER THINGS?

where are the slugs on YOUR Garden Gloves...?

ew!
get 'im off!

HOW TO DO IT...

Make a list of 25 things.
You'd love to Be doing more of
[or ANY of!] in Your life Right Now:

BIG...or small...

e.g., Have more meaning
to my work.

e.g; Ten minutes alone.

1.
2.
3.
4.
5.
6.
7.
8.
9.
10.
11.
12.
13.
14.
15.
16.
17.
18.
19.
20.
21.
22.
23.
24.
25.

Now...

How many of "those things" do you
actually let yourself do ?

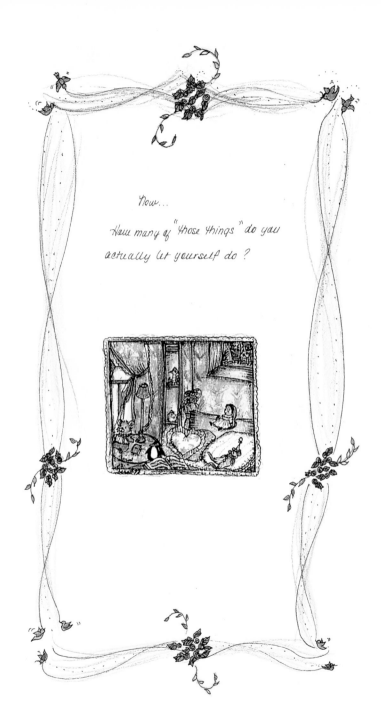

Balanced
Living
~ and eating and weighing ~
are
PROCESSES
~ not goals.

Working on

DEVELOPING
A
WORKABLE,
LIVABLE
process ...

is the goal
Unto itself.

We can only fit SO MUCH in our days...

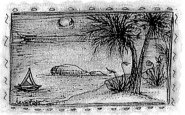

Why not keep it HAPPY & GOOD?

44

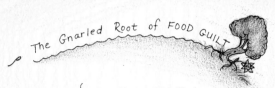

The Gnarled Root of FOOD GUILT

So not allow GUILT to
sabotage your efforts to unearth what
it is you really want to eat ~ even if it *is*
a "BAD" food.

"Bad" foods are novelty foods.
Take the "novelty" out of the foods, and they
become ordinary and not nearly so alluring. By

SYSTEMATICALLY INDULGING

in the foods you most
often reach for during a binge,
you are learning to eat more like a tree.
You are learning how to live with them at your
fingertips, the first step toward a more selective,
balanced approach to your consumption of them.

You are also balancing out those calories you
would ordinarily be denying yourself (and
binging on later), and you are making it SO MUCH
EASIER for your body to convert them into
useable energy.........................

Zap FOOD GUILT at the roots
(in YOUR MIND'S EYE)

Envision yourself eating your
most favorite foods ~ "bad," "good" & otherwise ~
in a calm way, in a pleasurable setting,
one bite at a time... SEE IT!

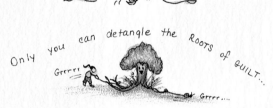

Only you can detangle the ROOTS of GUILT...

Grrrrr

Grrrr....

As long as you have eaten just what you felt like eating, in a fairly conscious manner (thinking about the taste and texture of the food and chewing each bite at a comfortable pace, not a rushed one), YOU HAVE TAKEN IN THOSE CALORIES WISELY.

Why?

Because you have filled a void that has the potential to grow much larger and deeper. And it will need a lot more to fill it later on, as we know all too well. By filling it NOW, as soon as the need or desire arises, you are ending it, and starting anew.

And then...
You are able to move on to the next task at hand. By addressing the INTERNAL NEED you have made the external environment a little bit better, because now that the craving is gone you can concentrate on the task at hand and do it more consciously ~ and, consequently, with a higher quality result.

That makes EVERYBODY happy!

Most importantly, you are getting into the HABIT of mindful, moderate, meaningful eating... the sure path to a weight your body AND mind will be at P E A C E with... forever!

Human beings, like trees, will always
instinctively attempt to keep the status quo,
within and without themselves. If a
tree goes too long without rain, it will
gobble up a huge amount of water, first
chance it gets. If we humans go too
long without food, we'll usually eat
almost anything that looks and tastes
edible, first chance we get. And, if we
say, "No," to the cheesecake we really crave
and want today, we may be setting
ourselves up for a binge on ANYTHING
sweet later.

Trees are at the mercy of Mother Nature,
for the most part, but we humans can fill
our needs as they arise. A habit of doing
so creates a moderate feeding pace, and
"grows" a moderate body weight along the way.

But what about "ALL THOSE OTHER THINGS"?
What happens when we deprive ourselves of
them?

—→

We
pig
out.

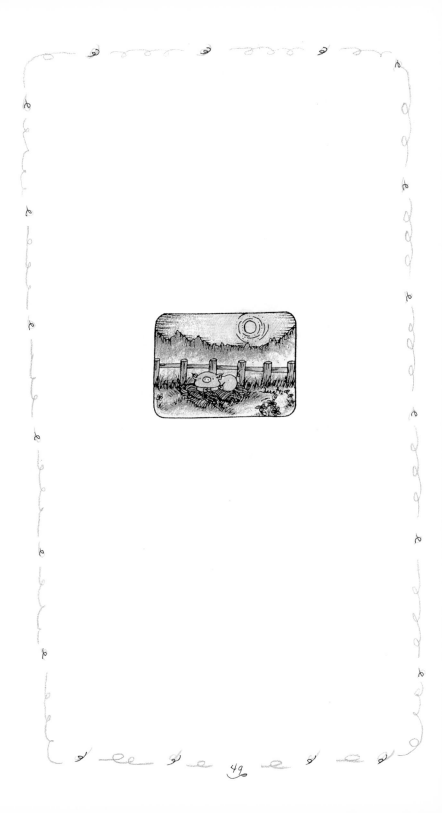

Perhaps the biggest misconception
"always skinny" people and society as
a whole perpetuate is that the overweight
are habitual overindulgers.

IN FACT, THE OPPOSITE IS TRUE:

Habitual
Overeaters
are
CHRONIC
DEPRIVERS...

...of "all those other things."

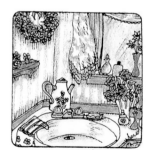

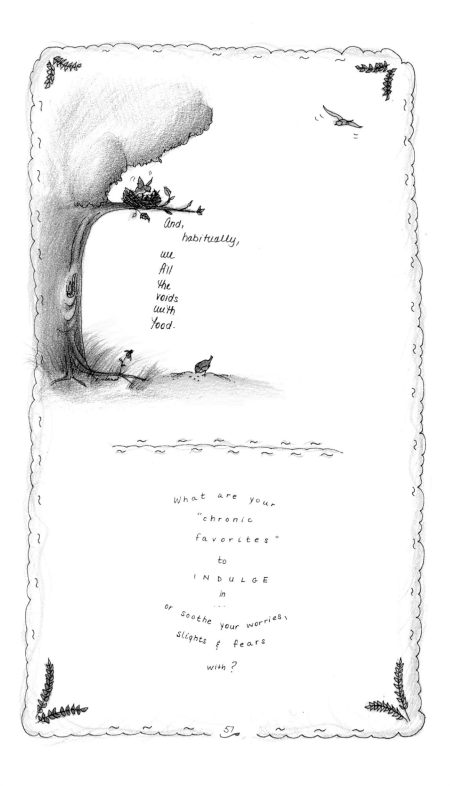

And,
habitually,
we
fill
the
voids
with
food.

What are your
"chronic
favorites"
to
INDULGE
in
...
or soothe your worries,
slights & fears

with?

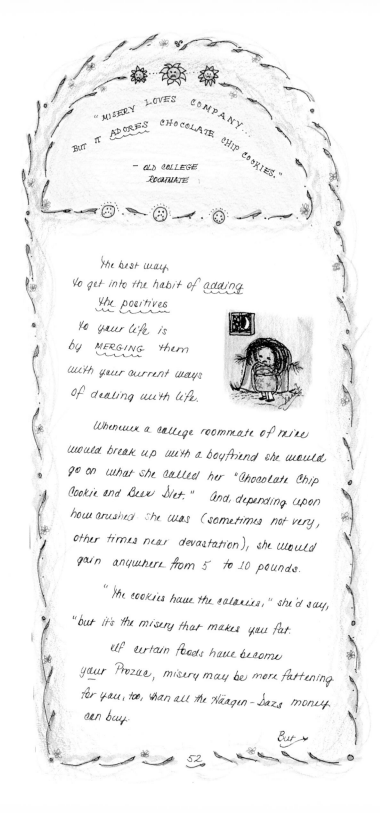

The best way
to get into the habit of adding
the positives
to your life is
by MERGING them
with your current ways
of dealing with life.

Whenever a college roommate of mine
would break up with a boyfriend she would
go on what she called her "Chocolate Chip
Cookie and Beer Diet." And, depending upon
how crushed she was (sometimes not very,
other times near devastation), she would
gain anywhere from 5 to 10 pounds.

"The cookies have the calories," she'd say,
"but it's the misery that makes you fat.
If certain foods have become
your Prozac, misery may be more fattening
for you, too, than all the Häagen-Dazs money
can buy.

But

MISERY

~ unfortunately ~

WILL ALWAYS BE OUT THERE !

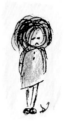

Just as we need rain and clouds to make the universe shine, so, too, do we need misery to keep us balanced and happy.

It's not Misery ~ but the manner in which you deal with it, if at all, that determines its calorie count for you. Are you stuffing down your sadness with food ? Or are you at the other end of the sadness spectrum : running away from it during too many minutes on your treadmill ?

Think about your own "Chocolate Chip Cookie and Beer Diet." What is it that you reach for most when you are sad, stressed, lonely, or angry? If it is food, what do the foods you reach for have in common ? Sweetness, creaminess, crunchiness, salt ? What does this food remind you of ? Do the chocolate chip cookies remind you of cozy afternoons after school, or holidays, or snow days at home in the kitchen with Grandma ?

Pinpoint the possible reasons for a particular binge food's allure.

And then, whatever you do, don't change a thing about what it is you eat.

Seriously...

ONCE YOU HAVE PINPOINTED

possible

connections

between the food and the

FEELING

it
provokes...

ADD SOMETHING ELSE THAT REMINDS YOU
OF THE SAME THING:

If it is a person you are missing, pick up a
good book or a movie to fill the lonely void
(while you eat the "cookies" and drink the "beer").

IF IT IS THE OLD COMFORTS
of
Home
that you crave,
wash your favourite blanket or comforter
with extra fabric softener
and snuggle in underneath it.

AND...

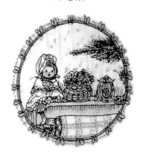

AS SILLY AS IT SOUNDS...

Never underestimate
the healing power of
a big,
fluffy
TEDDY BEAR
(or a big, fluffy pillow).

For Your Information

In case you don't already know:
Doggie breath doesn't
smell when it
touches human
tears
in a wet, slimy kiss.

The Important Thing is...

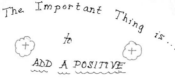

to

ADD A POSITIVE

(the comforter, the book, the bear)

BEFORE EVEN CONSIDERING TAKING SOMETHING

AWAY

(the cookies, the beer, the Häagen-Dazs).

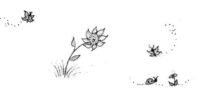

If you've ever started a lawn from seed,
    you know this all too well:
The only way to grow grass on stubborn
"bald spots" is to add dirt, add seed, add dirt,
add seed, until finally some begins to grow
and, eventually, anchors all the rest...

    Eventually, you may have added
        all three:
    (the comforter... the book ... the bear...)
By then, though, even the cookies, the beer,
and the ice cream don't compare to the
supreme, soul-warming comforts
        of

    all those other things....

(a good book, a sweet-smelling blanket,
    and a teddy bear to hug).

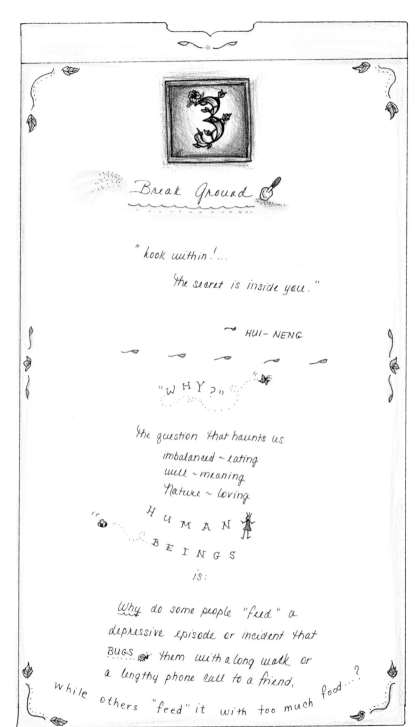

3

Break Ground

"Look within!...

the secret is inside you."

~ HUI-NENG

"WHY?"

the question that haunts us

imbalanced ~ eating
well ~ meaning
Nature ~ loving

H U M A N

B E I N G S

is:

Why do some people "feed" a depressive episode or incident that BUGS them with a long walk or a lengthy phone call to a friend, while others "feed" it with too much food...?

In order to get at the "bulb" of

H A B I T U A L

overeating

~ and the deprivation of "other things"

that eggs it on ~

we must dig a little, beneath the

surface

of what may look like a

"peaceful" existence ...

but in actuality may be one

D O M I N A T E D

by

boredom, stuffed anger, or

even

"automatic pilot."

WE MUST MAGNIFY

~ NOT

MODIFY ~

TO UNEARTH THOSE

DEFICIENCIES

of

"all those other things"

After all, before you start a garden,

it's always a good idea to do a soil test

to see what your dirt is lacking ....

For us humans,
a great way to "test the soil"
is
by keeping a

P E R S O N A L

Journal.

~ this does not have to be the
next great novel.

(although you may surprise
yourself
~ and the world at large ~
someday.!)

~ think of it first as a descriptive
little book of days, a personal

♥ B O O K
O F
Y O U ♥

If you are in the habit of
filling an unconscious need for

~ companionship

~ creativity

~ freedom in your
     daily day

...or a n y t h i n g except
a true hunger for

       F O O D ...

          with
      something
          to
       munch
         on,

your journal will help you to
pinpoint the REAL CAUSE
OF YOUR EMPTINESS INSIDE ~ so
it can soon get its proper fill.

In order to prepare
a site
for healthy, long-term

G R O W T H ;

you take a sampling
of
what you DO HAVE &
see what it is lacking

SO
that
YOU
CAN
ADD
WHAT
IT
IS
YOU
NEED
to right any imbalances.

You do not attempt to take the
"bad stuff" away ~ you ADD THE GOOD
and let Nature ameliorate
the rest.

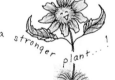

Kill the weeds with a stronger plant...!

This is called "overlapping the positives"

to squeeze out the negatives,

little by little.

In your journal, make a list
of several things you would like
to do during an ideal day.
REALLY THINK ABOUT THIS ... TRY TO
PICTURE IT IN YOUR MIND'S EYE.
You are :

1. Eating breakfast at a small,
   outdoor café.

2. Going for a long walk on the
   beach (hearing seagulls
   and waves crashing, feeling
   wet sand heavy between your
   toes...).

3. Working at a job you love,
   ♡♡♡ such as _____
   _____
   _____
   _____

4. Planning a vacation (...to:
   _____
   ..... and you'd pack : _____
   _____
   so that you could easily _____
   _____
   _____

5. Playing soccer with the kids,
   or tug-of-war, or House, or
   Barbie, or _____
   _____
   _____

etc... etc....

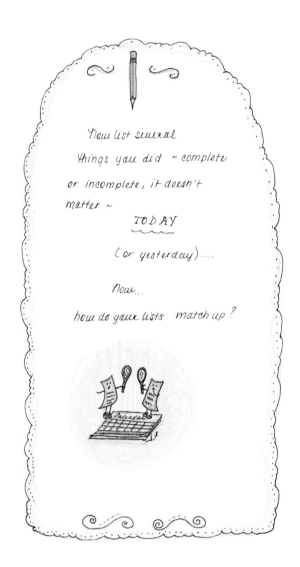

Now list several
things you did ~ complete
or incomplete, it doesn't
matter ~

TODAY

(or yesterday)....

Now...

how do your lists match up ?

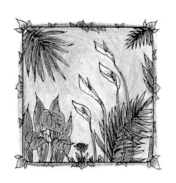

" The human mind
   always makes progress,
   but it is a progress in spirals. "

                    ～   MADAME DE STAËL

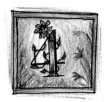

Dig Shallow & Wide

~ In your journal, make a list of 10
PEOPLE / ACTIVITIES / THINGS / PLACES
that are very valuable to you.

Compare these values to the list of
things you actually did today or yesterday.

Are you living in accordance with
what and who and where you value most
in this life?   If not:

· ~ you are not greedy

· ~ you are not lazy

· ~ you are not wrong

· ~ you are not ill equipped to do so...

YOU ARE DEPRIVING YOURSELF
of the personal growth and living truths
that you crave...

· ~ and you may be packing down
     those desires with too much food.

Not enough (of one or two or all "those other things")	+	Too much (chocolate chip COOKIE DOUGH ice cream... chips... burgers ... whatever)	=	A balance of sorts.

Like the tree that needs light, and air, and water, as well as the nutrients in the soil, so it is with us.

Expecting food alone to provide us with the physical and mental energy we need in order to function best is unrealistic and sets us up for failure time and time again. Food can only do so much.

It is up to us to find the energy sources around us, be they a good book, a hike in the woods, or a loud rock concert.

By beginning to see what we are lacking
we are beginning
to see what we
really & truly NEED
in this life ~
besides food.

But food IS important . . . .

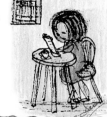

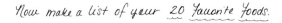

Now make a list of your <u>20</u> favorite foods.

How many did you eat yesterday?

Chances are, you ate either too much of one thing
or another, whether you meant to or not, and not enough
of something else.

The key to a moderate weight is moderate eating ~
NOT DEPRIVATION.

that means giving yourself the gift of

    ~ your favorite foods

    ~ your favorite pastimes

    ~ your most valued people

~ in the places you feel comfortable in ~

    a little bit, each and every day.

Like a tree, soaking up nutrients from the soil,
    a little bit at a time,
    each and every time
    it needs to.

TREE MYTH #1

When you plant
A TREE
in
your
yard...

Dig a deep hole.

~ ~ ~ ~ ~ ~ ~ ~

It seems like common sense to dig a deep hole the size of — or a little larger than — the root ball of a tree before you set it in the ground. On the contrary, most of a tree's roots grow in the top two feet of soil. As the tree grows, the roots stretch wider and wider, not deeper. If you've ever seen a tree that was uprooted in a storm, you know this. THE ROOTS FAN OUT IN SUNBURST FASHION, RATHER THAN IN A LONG, SPINDLY MASS.

The reason for this growth pattern of the roots of even the largest of trees is that the air, water, and nutrients that a tree needs are up there near the top. For this reason it is best to dig a hole that is SHALLOW AND W I D E This encourages the roots to STRETCH OUT IN SEARCH OF FOOD, SO THEY BECOME ADEPT AT FEEDING THE TREE FOR ITS MAXIMUM AMOUNT OF GROWTH AND STRENGTHENING THE TREE'S WIDE-SPANNING BRANCH SYSTEM THAT WILL GROW OVER TIME, REACHING FARTHER AND FARTHER EACH YEAR....

Without a healthy root system, a tree is just a log in dirt!

How does that relate to food & us?

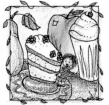

The roots of all eating are

THE HABITS THAT GOVERN IT.

The strength and longevity of these habits depend, too, on how far-reaching they stretch. The premise of unearthing the moderate eater in you is not to change who you are or thoroughly alter how you live. Deep digging, or eliminating or completely overhauling and bypassing the garden ground level, is not the way.

"UNEARTHING" MEANS BALANCING WHAT YOU WANT TO KEEP WITH THE POSITIVES YOU'VE ALWAYS WANTED TO ADD.

 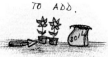

Moderate eating is based on balanced living. Healthier ways must lightly permeate MANY different aspects of THE LIFE YOU LEAD NOW.

Work on the HABIT of BALANCE in ALL areas of your life that could use it, and the eating habit will become one more root in the mass of the powerful, far-reaching approach of

M O D E R A T I O N

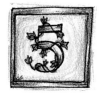

Prepare the Sail.

"Well must the ground
        be digg'd,
    and better dress'd,
New soil to make,
        and meliorate the rest."

~ JOHN DRYDEN

Now that we're beginning to see some deficiencies in the grand scheme of our lifestyles, it's time to plan a course of action.

(Notice we haven't even TOUCHED our plates yet... * whew *...What a refreshing approach to overcoming eating imbalances, no?).....

We've already begun SEEING more

~ of what's around us

~ of what we're up against

~ of what we are currently doing to accommodate that, and keep a "balance of sorts."

70

We have made progress
even if we only can remember to do
a little bit each and every day.
Preparing the soil, like all beginnings
of growth, takes time.

➝ It's usually done in small doses.

➝ It operates on ADDITION of the
good stuff ~ "all those other things" you
DO want more of in your life ~ not negative
worry about subtraction of "the bad stuff"
(like dessert and extra-pepperoni pizza,
stress on the job and too many chores at home).

"Preparing the soil " means creating
the FOUNDATION for BALANCE.

How do we create this
foundation for BALANCE ?

BALANCE =

All the good things
we can ADD
to our days

+

All the inevitable
"bad stuff"
out there.

Look at the tree.

Trees <u>eat</u> what they need
and <u>when</u> they need it. But they also
LET OUT THE STUFF THEY DON'T NEED.

Taking
in
soil nutrients,   Letting   a
sun ☼,   +   out   =   healthy,
CO_2 O_2 happy
&   tree
☁ rainwater

Before you even <u>think</u> of what
you "should" or "should not" be eating, take a
close look at how you let yourself <u>let out</u>
any <u>excess.</u>

In other words ...

Just as human bodies were meant
→ to eat (& enjoy it)
→ to breathe (fresh air from trees)
→ to love & belong (to a world bigger
than we are) ...

so, too, were we meant TO MOVE.

We need to move regularly ~ on a daily basis.

72

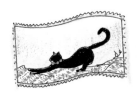

We need to stretch like old cats
(gently)...

We need to breathe deeply
(exhale first)
and
we need to
MOVE THE LIMBS WE WERE GIVEN.

If
the thought
of "exercise"
turns you off,
forget about that notion.
Right now it doesn't work for you
SO CONCENTRATE INSTEAD ON WHAT DOES.

Make Peace with your tastes.

You may abhor jogging.
THAT IS OKAY.

But ~
you may love long, leisurely walks
(or brisk 20-minute ones) to daydream or
to think about a problem that stumps you.

73

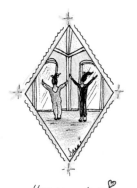

You may love ♡
going to a Yoga class with
a trusted friend, or reading a
great mystery on an exercise bicycle
in your bedroom ~ alone.

A good rule of thumb is,
if you can't picture yourself doing something
<u>willingly</u> every day for the next five years
(or almost every day), <u>DROP IT</u> and find something
better that you <u>CAN</u> stick with.

-¦- The key is to never stop "finding something."

Think of movement as
N O U R I S H M E N T
~ just as vital to your well-being as HUGS.
Journal time, venting and movement time ~ this
is <u>YOUR TIME</u>. And you have been depriving
yourself of these

✛ GOOD THINGS FOR YOUR SOUL ✛

for far too
long   74

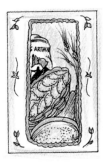

" A real gardener
is not a man who
cultivates flowers;
he is a man who cultivates
the soil. "

~ KAREL CAPEK
The Gardener's Year

Even if you begin with a 10-minute walk from
your car (parked at the other end of the parking lot)
to the grocery store doors, that is enough.

~ It is a step in the right direction, and even
small steps work over time..... 🌱

Our goal is only to cultivate the HABITS ~
the tendencies and inclinations and daily goings-on ~
that will heal us and bring us back to the
balanced environment that feeds us AS WHOLE
HUMAN BEINGS.

Even 10-minute walks ~ which don't
seem like much ~ count.

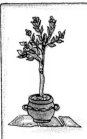

TREE MYTH #2:

Plant the tree in heavily amended soil.

Tree experts used to recommend adding a lot of "tree goodies" to the dirt you transplant a tree into, deep, rich soil heavy with nutrients and organic matter.

This presents a problem: a tree whose roots never have to leave the dig hole in order to look for food doesn't have the opportunity to develop a wide-reaching root system. Planting a tree in special soil is like feeding and raising a wild animal. If the animal becomes dependent on you for food and shelter it would starve if suddenly cast back out on its own. While instinct would help it over time, it may take a while for the animal to tap back into these natural inclinations. In the meantime, it may not have the fully developed skills needed for survival that other animals have that were out in the wild all along.

This is precisely what may happen to you if you simply switch to prepackaged diet foods without changing the habits that distanced you from your natural weight ideal in the first place. The amount of fat in the food has changed, but the nutritional value hasn't, and neither have the habits. You may still eat mindlessly, or too quickly, or not in accordance with your cravings. And you may not be leaving the table satisfied and energized for the next task at hand ~ definitely not an "ideal" you can live with for long.

Strong, far-reaching roots anchor a tree in the wildest of storms; all-pervasive habits of moderation will carry you through any buffet line comfortably, so that you can leave the restaurant satisfied ~ neither bloated nor feeling deprived.

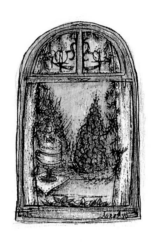

"Each man must look to himself
to teach him the meaning of life.
It is not something discovered:
it is something molded."

~ ANTOINE DE SAINT~ EXUPERY

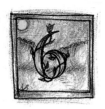

Add Organic Matter.

(Don't ~~change~~... simply enrich the soil you have to work with...
TODAY !)

~ ~ ~ ~ ~

Without water, a tree will die.
We need water, too.

Our bodies are composed of the same
percentage of water ~ about 65% ~ as the earth.
And, just as ponds evaporate and rivers run dry,
so do we.

Add water 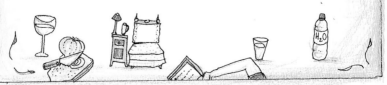 ~ even if only Dixie Cups
full, here and there, at first ~ to your daily
routine :

~ as you prepare dinner
~ beside your bed at night
~ beside your elbow at work or home
~ in a small bottle in the car

Drinking a steady stream of water
throughout the day
keeps your cells happy,
your system regular, and your
stomach less bloated over time. It
keeps your skin moist (but not TOO), your
hair shiny, and your appetite even.

⁓ WATER and MOVEMENT are
the 2 chief ingredients we need to live a
balanced life, from the inside out. They
are the "organic matter" I refer to.

Remember...

developing the habit of moderation is
about ADDING
⁓ not taking away ⁓
because adding "the good stuff"
makes cutting back or eliminating
"the bad stuff"
a nonconcern

It just naturally balances out.

Because, as you add movement and water to your day,
as you add fresh foods
to what you already eat,
as you get out the "stuff" that,
up until now, may have been "strangling
your roots," an EQUILIBRIUM emerges, and...

suddenly you wake up
and realize how special
you really are
and how long you've waited
to treat yourself well
and how much you deserve
to care for yourself
by nourishing your every need
       every single day

~ even just a little bit.

Like root food, this nourishment
feeds the whole you, from the INSIDE.

And suddenly the outside
~ the uncontrollable climate ~
looks a whole lot better...

because you make it that way.

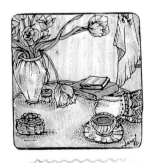

Moderate eating is not eating
with a fat-free crutch. It's QUALITY over
quantity eating, quality meaning exactly
what your body and your mind want and
need to eat and to live well.

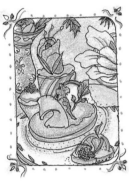

As you address more and more
of your cravings, even for "junk," begin to
add some mental fuel to your commitment
toward personal wellness, even if you are
not quite ready to change the way you eat.
Simply MOVE MORE , DRINK MORE WATER ,
and keep listening to what your feelings,
your taste buds, and your body are telling
you.

So these things ANYWAY.

An exercise in conscious eating...

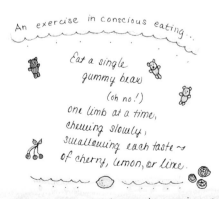

Eat a single
gummy bear
(oh no!)
one limb at a time,
chewing slowly,
swallowing each taste ~
of cherry, lemon, or lime.

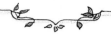

TREE MYTH #3:

Prune the tree as soon as you plant it.

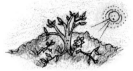

Experts used to say you should cut away about one-third of a tree's branches soon after transplanting. The theory was that by doing so, most of the tree's energy would go into developing strong roots.

On the contrary, if you remove the branches, a tree will attempt to right the imbalance by putting its energy into replacing the lost limbs. The result? Certainly not stronger <u>roots</u> ~ the lifelines of any tree.

Experts nowadays recommend pruning away only the dead branches and allowing the tree to settle in and grow for at least the first year after transplanting. Only then should low-hanging branches be pruned sparingly.

Diets suggest a similar theory: lose the weight and the habits ~ the lifelines of any permanent weight loss ~ will come naturally to maintain it. For most of us, however, the opposite is true. The habits ~ the roots ~ have to come first. Then all food is "safe." All eating situations are "safe."

Forget about the diet part of weight loss, and skip over to maintenance. Once you are at your ideal body weight, how are you going to keep it? That's what healthy eating is all about: THE PROCESS UNIQUE AND NATURAL TO YOU THAT WILL GET YOU TO AND KEEP YOU AT YOUR IDEAL WEIGHT FOR GOOD.

> "Your proper concern is alone
> the action of duty, not the fruits of the action.
> Cast then away all desire and fear for the fruits,
> and perform your duty."
>
> ~ The Bhagavad Gita

The Thin GREEN Line

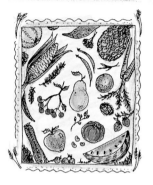

Think of FOOD CALORIES as units of strength.

Along with eating exactly the foods you crave, and eating them as often as possible in a calm, nurturing environment, the best way to increase the QUALITY of your eating habits is to increase the AMOUNT and FREQUENCY of eating GREEN:

↝ adding an apple to your quick lunch sandwich
(try it before the sandwich as an "appetizer"!)

↝ drinking a V-8 with breakfast

 ↝ grabbing a small bag of raw baby carrots to munch on as your stomach growls in traffic

Think of FRUITS & VEGGIES as "in-betweens" in your Favorite Foods Days
↝ every day! ↝

83

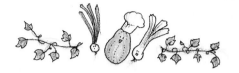

Become a veggie connoisseur:

~ Shop organic (i.e., pesticide-free) whenever possible (and support your local farmer as often as you can!)

~ Experiment with classic vegetable-based recipes on your day off, if you like to cook (yet another relaxing outlet for many):

Try: ~ Fresh tomato sauce

~ Ratatouille

~ Eggplant parmesan
(bake it for less mess ~ greasy fat splatters ~ instead of frying)

~ An assortment of root vegetables (carrots, potatoes, leeks, zucchini squash & garlic; sweet potatoes, turnips, beets & onion...). Choose your favorites, cut them up, and toss them in a good olive oil (and bread crumbs for a toasted crunch). Roast in a hot (450°F or higher) oven till tender.

 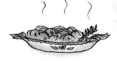 ? ? ? Enjoy!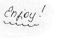

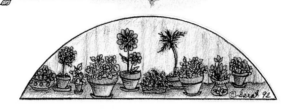

Learn about fresh herbs:

~ how to grow them

~ how to cook with them

~ how to use them as natural remedies

~ how to make a beautiful herbal wreath
or sachet to feed your other senses, too.

When you get used to
the taste
of fresh herbs
on your food,
no other seasoning can compare ~ extra salt,
extra butter, extra special sauce... none can
measure up to:

~ fresh parsley and lemon on fish
  (with freshly ground peppercorns)

~ fresh basil leaves on a sandwich

~ fresh rosemary on chicken

~ fresh dill in a new potato salad

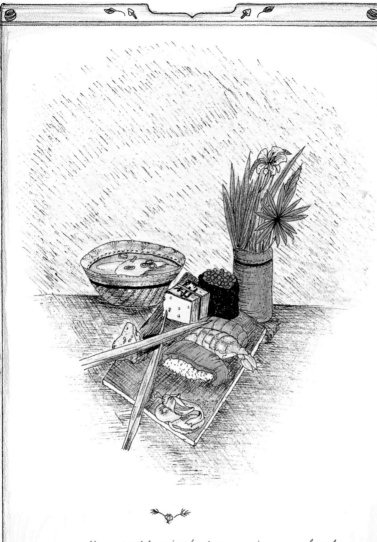

You could simply browse in your local bookstore at the myriad of beautiful cookbooks for tips. Check out television cooking shows for ideas and excellent instruction, not to mention entertainment. Or take a class, alone or with a friend.

Even if you're not ready to do much yet, just LOOK.

Looking is a BIG first step

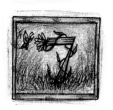

Mulch to Protect.

Moderate eating requires a somewhat balanced environment in which to thrive. And that takes <u>your attention</u>.

Let a garden grow unattended far too long, and weeds are bound to pop up (sometimes overnight!). But if you protect the tender soil with a light layer of mulch, and pull a weed or two every day, it's bound to do just fine.

Everything you have read about in this book is "the mulch to protect."

Daily time for you:

- ~ to think
- ~ to move
- ~ to write in your journal
- ~ to read something enriching to <u>your soul.</u>
- ~ little pieces of what's already there, mixed anew with what you may have forgotten...

...Like a steaming bowl of blueberry-studded oatmeal on A CHILLY WINTER MORNING!

~ the excitement of waiting for a
    creamy dessert ...

        (a <u>necessity</u>, on occasion !)

~ the nip in the air when spring turns
    into summer into fall ...

        (walk briskly and
        "eat up" that air !)

~ the security of bringing your own
    lunch ...

        (reminds you of Home,
        even at Work)

~ the thrill of donning a bathing suit
    and running straight into the
    ocean, on the first beach day of
    the summer ...

        (nobody's body is your
        body's ideal ~ who
        cares ? ~ life is too
        short to miss out on
        <u>FUN</u> !!!)

~ all the things you remember with
    warmth and good feeling from
    your childhood ~ food-wise and
    otherwise ~ and all of the things
    you treasure as an adult.

This is what makes ~ and keeps ~

    a balanced body
    a peaceful mind
    in a moderate, happy life ... !

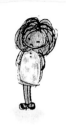

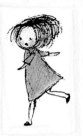

Perfection is not the goal.
Getting back to the True You is.

And that does not require a high-wire
walk of restriction nor does it require
sharp-eyed attention to every detail
of your day.

But it does require your
ATTENDANCE

⁓ regularly

⁓ and unconditionally.

You deserve this ~
You are the only "YOU" this earth
has. And like each tiny bird and
every sapling that sprouts, you are
precious to us all.

Please, take care
of
our
"You."

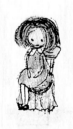

SHOWCASE YOUR TALENT

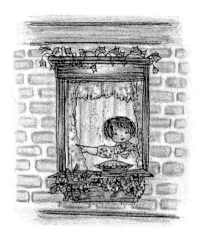

...Whether it be baking a pie...
or talking to an unhappy
friend...
or washing a mean dish...
or
building a birdhouse
or
peeling an apple
all in one skin
or
making your little nephew giggle,
it is essential to us all
on
Planet Earth....

How else can we taste it, enjoy it,
live better because of it ~
YOU ARE THE ONLY GIVER OF YOU...
Please don't deprive us of YOU!

Eating
like a tree
is merely a
M E T A P H O R
(or is it a simile ???)
for taking in all the things
that you require for
a lifestyle amenable to your
nature
(your
uniqueness,
in body
in mind
in spirit).
Always
note
how
you
feel...
what you want...
and how best to utilize all that
for the greatest good, so that the
environment you nourish gives back to you
in turn, and you perpetuate the cycle by
living and caring (for you) at your inherent best.

That's what 'eating like a tree'
is all about.

Now pick up your "spade" (your pen, your journal,
YOUR OWN THOUGHTS & TIME TO THINK THEM) and go
underground, to the roots, to the Source. As you get closer
to your personal truths ~ about food, about what your
life is lacking (or not), and about your feelings for yourself ~
you will be in the PROCESS of getting closer to your own
personal weight, eating, living, and loving Eden.

V

HOW TO EAT LIKE A TREE

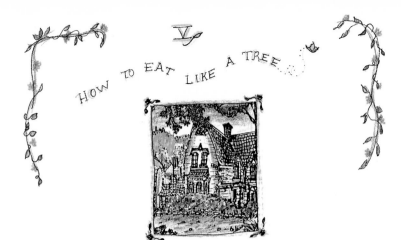

"Let me look upward
into the towering oak and know
that it grew great and strong
because it grew slowly
and well."

~ ORIN L. CRAIN

Taking in all you need and
letting out all that you do not is a
DAILY PROCESS. Following are some
ways that you may choose to apply
the principles of this book to your
daily life.

Before you get
out of bed
tomorrow morning,
lie in your drowsiness
and let it show you
from the inside
the You
you want to be:
your living ideal ♥

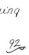

Let
the garden,
or any part of
N A T U R E
that you help to create,
BE YOUR GUIDE...

Raise it as best you know how
and it will reward you
with nourishment
from the inside out.

listen
to your
"gut"
feelings.
They are usually right,
and hold their own rewards.

Do not
be afraid
to plateau
once in a while.
Plan for it.
Even the wildest
of oceans are placid
at times.

Turn
to the ocean
or the lake
or the rain
to wash away your hurt.
(A warm shower is nice, too...
or a run through the sprinkler...)

If
you sense a
food binge beckoning,
decide what you'd most
like to eat, and buy them
in single or double serving sizes.
Then eat them, as slowly as possible.
But before you buy them, decide on
a KIND thing to do for yourself
   AFTER YOU EAT.

Eat... then treat.

This one's hard... ♡ ... but practice will pay off!

Practice
crying in private,
so that your tears
can release
the frustration
instead
of
the
act
of
eating.

94

HOW TO EAT LIKE A TREE

The most beautiful
of flowers
take time
to grow.

Give yourself time
in all that you do,
and
you, too,
will blossom.

Know
that
H A P P I N E S S
is
not
always
rational.

Never forget: inside every
failure
is the seed
~ sometimes quite small ~
of a wonderful success
waiting for you
in disguise.

Sometimes you have to dig around in the dirt a while
before you can find it! 95

HOW TO EAT LIKE A TREE...

Make a list
of 10 things
~ You Do Well
~ You Like About Yourself
~ You Like About Your Body
~ You Like About Your Life
as it is
Today.

⭐ ⭐ ⭐

Simply **KNOW** that it will be Okay...

(whatever your "it" is).

The next time
you're outside
and the wind blows,
close your eyes
and
Just **FEEL** it

Move
to stretch
muscles
that were meant
to be moved.

Move so that your mind can be more
at
peace.

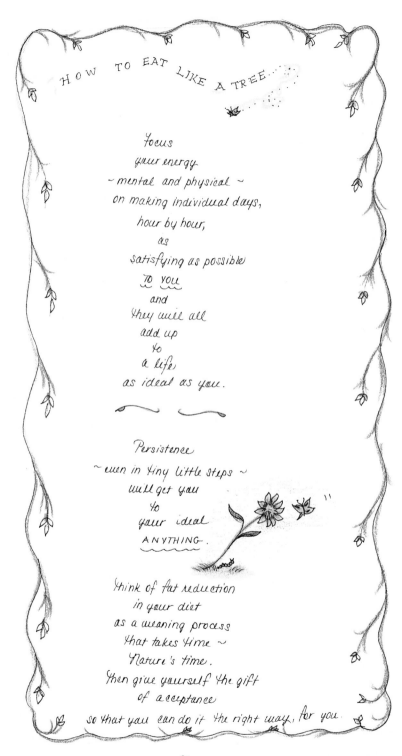

Focus
your energy
~ mental and physical ~
on making individual days,
hour by hour,
as
satisfying as possible
TO YOU
and
they will all
add up
to
a life,
as ideal as you.

Persistence
~ even in tiny little steps ~
will get you
to
your ideal
ANYTHING.

Think of fat reduction
in your diet
as a weaning process
that takes time ~
Nature's time.
Then give yourself the gift
of acceptance
so that you can do it the right way, for you.

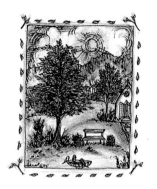

"Convince me that you
have a seed there,
and I am prepared
to expect wonders."

~ HENRY DAVID THOREAU
<u>Faith in a Seed</u>

VI

PLANTING NEW SEEDS...

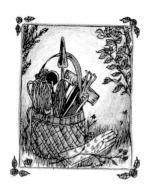

Nature plants her own seeds.

We know this from experience: a tiny mimosa tree sprouts up on the corner of the lawn, its mother tree clear across the yard; a rose of Sharon seemingly multiplies of its own accord; wildflowers reappear from year to year, as little birds and big breezes scatter their leftover seeds.

And so it is with us.

As you add little healthy, NURTURING tendencies, gestures, hobbies, and s i n g l e m o m e n t s of awareness to your average day, something wonderful occurs, quite naturally:

They multiply...

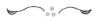

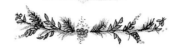

⌁ As you learn to set aside 10 minutes
(or more!) to jot down your thoughts or to doodle
in your journal, you realize you look forward
to that time of quiet introspection. You begin
to hear your own inner voice, perhaps for
the first time in your entire adult life...

⌁ As you begin to eat more consciously, you start
to see that you've been force-feeding taste buds you
just don't have, and ignoring those you really do.
You may realize that hunger was really thirst
(keep drinking those little Dixie cups of water
throughout the day); you begin to discern a craving
for chocolate cake from a yen for a good cry; you
begin to recognize a real satisfaction from the
creaminess of a bright, cooked carrot; and the ability
to _stop after just one_ seems to emerge by itself,
as the voids that need filling slowly get their
proper fill.

And, finally, as you begin to plant these
new seeds of POSITIVITY , you see how much energy
was once wasted on self-defeat and negativity., and
you embark upon the most wonderful journey of
True Growth that there is:

The Discovery of You.

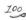

MODERATE LIVING

like
all
lasting
growth

is a process.

It's one of internally generated
power, spurred on by a nurturing environment.

Trees cannot move themselves if planted
in the wrong spot. We humans CAN. But we also
must recognize when it is WE who must adapt to what
it is we were given.

Decide where you want to be in this life,
no matter how dreamy, and begin to "eat" to get
there ... food-wise, self-education-wise, and
environment-wise.

Your Life is your Garden

How you choose to foster its growth
is certainly up to you. But remember, there's
a world of natural (i.e., human and other
living) resources out there to help you,
so that we all can live well, and contribute
that wellness to each other...

Just as we were meant to,
from the very beginning . . . . .

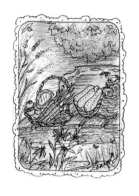

"The more one gardens,
the more one learns."

~ VITA SACKVILLE - WEST

~ Self-realization is a lifelong process ~
of growth fostered by self-love. A great way
to spur us on in the beginning and throughout
our journey to eating and living equilibrium
is via self-education; the words of others can
be nutrition for the soul....

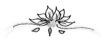

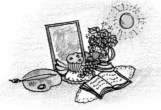

Nourishment for the Body

Blonz, Edward R., Ph.D. <u>The Really Simple, No Nonsense</u> <u>Nutrition Guide</u>. Berkeley, CA : Conari Press, 1993.

Margen, Sheldon, M.D., and the Editors of the University of California at Berkeley Wellness Letter. <u>The Wellness</u> <u>Encyclopedia of Food and Nutrition : How to Buy, Store, and</u> <u>Prepare Every Variety of Fresh Food</u>. New York : Rebus, 1992.

Nourishment for the Whole You

UNEARTHING THE IDEAL YOU :

Bennett, Hal Zina. <u>Follow Your Bliss</u>. New York : Avon Books, 1990.

Gawain, Shakti. <u>Return to the Garden : A Journey of Self-Discovery</u>. San Rafael, CA : New World Library, 1989.

UNEARTHING FALSE VISIONS :

Freedman, Rita. <u>BodyLove : Learning to Like Our Looks ~ and Ourselves</u>. New York : Harper and Row, 1988.

Wolf, Naomi. <u>The Beauty Myth : How Images of Beauty are Used Against Women</u>. New York : William Morrow, 1991.

~UNEARTHING WHAT YOU WERE *Really* MEANT TO DO:

Bradley, Margaret E. *Your Natural Gifts*. 1972. McLean, VA: EPM Publications, 4lne., 1986.

Fritz, Robert. *The Path of Least Resistance: Learning to Become the Creative Force in Your Own Life.* New York: Fawcett Columbine / Ballantine, 1989.

Winter, Barbara J. *Making a Living Without a Job.* New York: Bantam, 1993.

~UNEARTHING SELF-CARE:

Kinder, Dr. Melvyn. *Going Nowhere Fast: Step Off Life's Treadmill and Find Peace of Mind.* New York: Prentice Hall Press, 1990.

Robinson, Bryan, Ph.D. *Overdoing it: How to Slow Down and Take Care of Yourself.* Deerfield Beach, FL: Health Communications, 4lne., 1992.

~UNEARTHING THE SITE OF YOUR NATURAL EATING IDEAL:

Moran, Victoria. *The Love-Powered Diet.* San Rafael, CA: New World Library, 1992.

Moyers, Bill. *Healing and the Mind.* New York: Doubleday, 1993.

~UNEARTHING PERSONAL VALUES:

Nearing, Helen and Scott. *Living the Good Life: Helen and Scott Nearing's Sixty Years of Self-Sufficient Living.* 1954. New York: Schocken Books, 1970.

Briggs, Dorothy Corkille. *Celebrate Your Self: Enhancing Your Own Self-Esteem.* New York: Doubleday, 1977.

Sanford, Linda Tschirhart, and Mary Ellen Donovan. *Women and Self-Esteem.* New York: Anchor/Doubleday, 1984.

Steinem, Gloria. *Revolution From Within: A Book of Self-Esteem.* 1992. Boston: Little, Brown and Company, 1993.

UNEARTHING DREAMS

Waitley, Denis. *Seeds of Greatness: The Ten Best-Kept Secrets of Success.* Old Tappan, NJ: Revell, 1983.

Walters, J. Donald. *Money Magnetism: How to Attract What You Need When You Need It.* Nevada City, CA: Crystal Clarity Publishers, 1992.

Weider, Marcia. *Making Your Dreams Come True: A Plan for Easily Discovering and Achieving the Life You Want.* New York: Mastermedia Limited, 1993.

and, first and finally:

You. *Your Personal Journal.* Wherever You Are: Whatever You Unearth and Add to Your Current Life, Anytime.

"Most of the shadows of this life
are caused by standing in one's own sunshine."

~ RALPH WALDO EMERSON

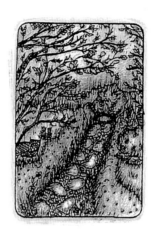

"And the end
of all our exploring
will be to arrive
where we started
And know the place
for the first time."

~ T.S. ELIOT
Four Quartets